ANTI INFLMMATORY MEAL PREP FOR BEGINNERS

DR. PENNY WATSON

Copyright © 2023 by Dr. Penny Watson

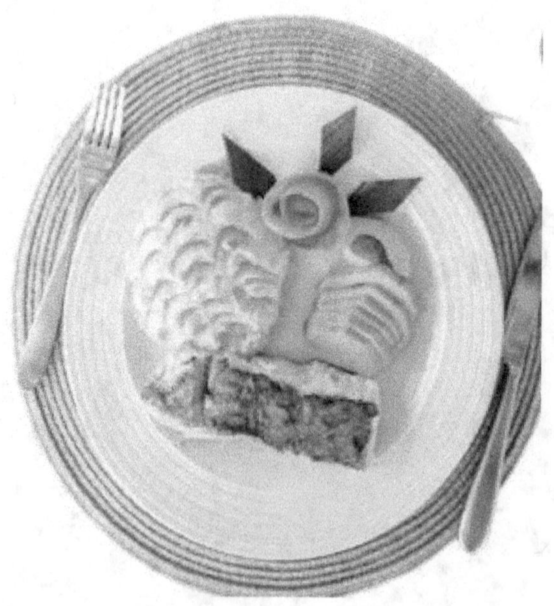

TABLE OF CONTENTS

INTRODUCTION...7

CHAPTER ONE 9

8 Caribbean Cultural Foods For Combating Inflammation.... 9

Reduce Inflammation and Joint Pain With Natural Anti Inflammatory Foods 16

CHAPTER TWO 23

Top 5 Anti Inflammatory Foods (Best List)........................ 23

Anti Inflammatory Food And Fruits To Reduce Joint Pain For Better Results... 27

Other Anti Inflammatory Foods 30

Anti Inflammatory Foods to Add to Your Diet 31

CHAPTER THREE 39

Anti Inflammatory Foods   How Important Are They In Our Life?... 39

Anti Inflammatory Diet: What To Know 41

CHAPTER FOUR.. **51**

Other Health Benefits of An Anti Inflammatory Diet.......... 51

12 Easy Ways To Reduce Inflammation Overnight 57

CHAPTER FIVE **67**

Anti Inflammatory Meal Prep Recipes 67

1. Turmeric Chickpea Quinoa Bowl 67

2. Salmon and Asparagus Sheet Pan Meal 68

3. Anti Inflammatory Green Smoothie 69

4. Mediterranean Chickpea Salad 70

5. Roasted Vegetable and Quinoa Bowl 71

6. Spinach and Quinoa Stuffed Bell Peppers 72

7. Berry and Walnut Overnight Oats 73

8. Roasted Garlic and Lemon Broccoli 74

9. Cilantro Lime Shrimp Bowl 75

10. Berry Spinach Salad with Almond Dressing 76

11. Baked Salmon with Dill and Turmeric 77

12. Quinoa and Lentil Salad 78

13. Spiced Sweet Potato Soup 79

14. Greek Quinoa Salad 80

15. Almond and Blueberry Protein Bars 81

16. Mediterranean Chickpea and Quinoa Bowl 82

17. Turmeric and Ginger Carrot Soup 83

18. Mixed Berry Chia Pudding 84

19. Roasted Brussels Sprouts and Butternut Squash 85

20. Green Tea and Ginger Infused Water 86

21. Mediterranean Quinoa Salad 87

22. Anti Inflammatory Turmeric Tea 88

23. Broccoli and Red Lentil Soup 89

Ingredients: 89

24. Spiced Chickpea and Vegetable Curry 90

25. Anti Inflammatory Berry Smoothie 91

26. Lemon Garlic Shrimp and Asparagus 92

27. Cabbage and Kale Slaw 93

28. Turmeric and Ginger Baked Chicken 94

29. Anti Inflammatory Berry Chia Jam 95

30. Spinach and Feta Stuffed Chicken Breast 96

CONCLUSION **99**

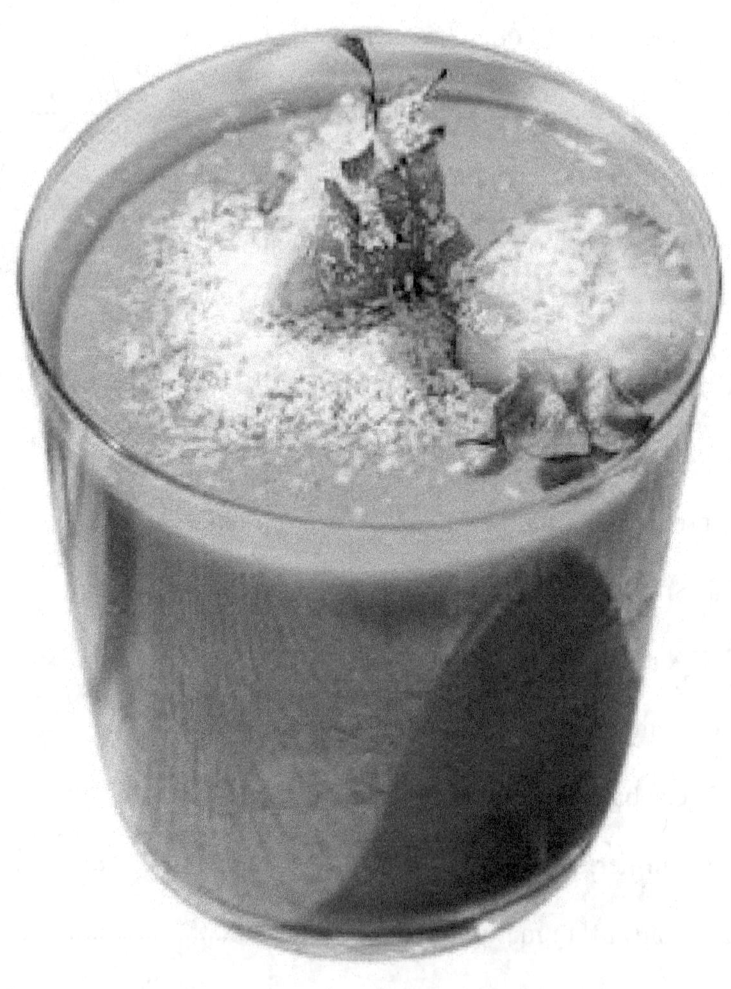

INTRODUCTION

There is no one anti inflammatory diet, rather, there are diets designed around foods that are believed to decrease inflammation and which shun foods that aggravate the inflammatory processes.

Many antiinflammatory diets are based around whole grains, legumes, nuts, seeds, fresh vegetables and fruits, wild fish and seafood, grass fed lean turkey and chicken which are thought to aid in the bodies healing of inflammation.

They exclude foods that are thought to trigger inflammation such as refined grains, wheat, corn, full fat dairy, red meat, caffeine, alcohol, peanuts, sugar, saturated and trans saturated fats.

The common foundation of anti inflammatory diets is the belief that low grades of inflammation are the precursor and/or antagonizer to many chronic diseases. Once removed, the body can begin healing itself.

Inflammation is a localized reaction of tissue to injury, whether caused by bacteria or viral infection, trauma, chemicals, heat or other phenomenon that causes irritation. The 'irritation' causes the tissues within the body to release multiple substances that cause changes within the tissues. This complex response is called inflammation. Inflammation is characterized by such symptoms that include:

1. Vasodilatation of the local blood vessels resulting in excess local blood flow.

2. Increases in the permeability of the capillaries with leakage of large quantities of fluid into the interstitial spaces.

3. Clotting of the fluid in the interstitial spaces due to excess amounts of fibrinogen and other proteins leaking from the capillaries.

4. Relocation of granulocytes and monocytes into the tissue in large quantities.

5. Swelling of the tissue cells.

CHAPTER ONE

8 Caribbean Cultural Foods For Combating Inflammation

Inflammation is the body's natural response to injury and infection.

However, chronic inflammation — which may be influenced by diet, inadequate sleep, and high stress levels — is linked to overweight and obesity, insulin resistance, diabetes, heart disease, and cancer. Fortunately, studies have shown that some cultural foods common to the Caribbean region, as well as overall lifestyle habits, fight inflammation.

Here are 8 anti inflammatory foods common to the Caribbean and its diasporas.

1. Cocoa and dark chocolate

The Caribbean has a longstanding history of producing quality cocoa products, with the Trinidad & Tobago Fine Cocoa Company among the oldest.

Flavanols — antioxidants found in cocoa products — have anti inflammatory properties that may protect blood vessel health, potentially reducing your risk of developing heart disease and stroke. They may also improve exercise performance and recovery.

Furthermore, flavanol rich cocoa and dark chocolate guard against blood vessel damage from oxidative stress, which occurs with age and in people who smoke, by increasing nitric oxide production Nitric oxide is a compound that may reduce inflammation and support healthy blood flow.

The higher the percentage of cocoa that dark chocolate contains, the more flavanols and greater antioxidant properties it has — although it may be slightly less palatable, as high percentages of cocoa increase bitterness.

2. West Indian cherry (acerola)

West Indian cherry, also called acerola (Malpighia emarginata), is lauded for the high levels of ascorbic acid (vitamin C) that it.

One cup (98 grams) of this fruit contains 1,650 mg of vitamin C.

That's 18 to 22 times the daily intake recommendation of 75 mg for women and 90 mg for men

Vitamin C fights inflammation by reducing the number of free radicals — the by products of metabolism — in the body.

Current research is exploring its potential to reduce the risk of developing some cancers.

3. Pimento pepper

Peppers of the capsicum family, including pimento pepper (Capsicum annum), contain phytochemical compounds that may have antioxidant and anti inflammatory properties.

These include flavonoids, quercetin, alkaloids, carotenoids, and capsaicinoids

In animal studies, capsaicin — the spicy component of mild and hot peppers — reduced the release of pro inflammatory compounds by adipose tissue in rats with obesity.

 It also reduced cell damage in the guts of However, human research is needed.

The pimento pepper is related to the habanero pepper (Capsicum chinense), but it's less spicy. It's traditionally used to add flavor to myriad cooked dishes, including stews and soups.

4. Red sorrel

Red sorrel (Hibiscus sabdariffa), also called roselle, is a mainstay in traditional medicine.

Both animal and human studies found that red sorrel may lower blood pressure and cholesterol. It may also reduce body weight, insulin resistance, and markers of inflammation.

One study determined that the plant is a good candidate to investigate for its role as an herbal supplement for cancer prevention and treatment. More human clinical trials are needed, though.

The benefits of red sorrel may be attributed to its abundance of anthocyanins, in addition to other polyphenols, and hibiscus acids

Roselle tea is quite popular as a hot or cold beverage.

In the Caribbean, fresh and dried leaves of the plant are primarily used to make the traditional Christmastime drink sorrel juice.

5. Passion fruit

Extracts of the Passiflora family, including passion fruit (Passiflora edulis), have long been used in herbal medicines to treat anxiety and convulsive disorders

It contains potent anti inflammatory and antioxidant compounds, such as flavonoids, piceatannol, and triterpenoids, which may lower blood pressure, cholesterol, and high blood sugar levels

One study found that piceatannol extract from passion fruit improved insulin sensitivity, blood pressure, and heart rate in men with overweight. However, it didn't have the same effect on women with moderate weight or women with overweight More human research is needed.

Passion fruit is tart, but you can eat it raw or make it into juice or lilikoi jelly, a staple breakfast food in Hawaiian culture.

6. Curcumin (turmeric)

Curcumin may have anti inflammatory health benefits that protect brain health and fight against diabetes, heart disease, bowel disease, arthritis, obesity related inflammation, and cancer.

Curcumin is the active compound in turmeric that provides the spice with its antioxidant and anti inflammatory properties.

Combining curcumin with piperine, the active ingredient in black pepper, may enhance your body's curcumin absorption, making more of this powerful compound available to reduce inflammation.

In the Caribbean, turmeric is commonly added to dishes prepared with Indian spices, including curry and geera (ground cumin).

7. Ginger

Ginger is common in cooked foods and hot beverages throughout the Caribbean.

Its major active components — 6 gingerol and 6 shogaol — improve enzyme pathways related to obesity induced inflammation, rheumatoid arthritis, aging, and neurocognitive diseases

Studies show that whole ginger extract, or 6 shogaol, may reduce chronic lung inflammation. One in vitro study suggests that it could be used as a therapeutic treatment for asthma in the future

However, more human research is needed.

Ginger may have anti inflammatory benefits that protect against rheumatoid arthritis, aging, and neurodegenerative diseases.

It's being studied for potential use as an asthma treatment.

8. Cinnamon

Cinnamon is well known for its role in reducing blood sugar

Rats on a high fat diet supplemented with polyphenol extracts from cinnamon bark experienced a reduction in inflammation from adipose tissues and improved insulin resistance

However, human studies have yielded conflicting results.

For instance, one review showed that supplementation with cinnamon significantly reduced most markers of inflammation

But on the other hand, two clinical trials in people with type 2 diabetes showed that cinnamon supplementation reduced cholesterol levels, but inconsistently reduced markers of inflammation.

More research is needed, but studies suggest that cinnamon may be used as an adjunct to conventional medicine to combat inflammation.

Reduce Inflammation and Joint Pain With Natural Anti Inflammatory Foods

We know it does work; you can start the body's healing process by targeting an effected area with essential nutrients.

As I have written several articles about health in general, I can confirm about my own issues concerning arthritis and joint pain that effected several parts of my body, which I have cured myself and for some years now have been pain free.

This is a matter of making your own decision to turn your life around and take things in a new direction. I know it is possible and achievable, because I've been there and done it. I also know what the biggest obstacle is for most, I see this again and again; it's the one thing that stops people succeeding to take control of their own health is this starting.

As with inflammation, joint pain, cartilage, we've been told once cartilage cells are damaged it is too late and the only option would be an operation. Yet there is strong prove that cartilage cells can repair themselves and restore the vital connection tissues around them.

A healthy cartilage is about 70% water and it must stay hydrated to function properly and to stay free of pain. Glucosamine will keep this water in the cartilage.

Drawing nutrient rich fluid from the body to repair and keep the joints healthy and free of pain.

That means many times there is no joint replacement surgery required; just a simple, harmless infrared light treatment can stop the pain in a matter of weeks. This is why an operation should only be done as the very last option and only if everything else has failed.

Drugs are not able to solve the root cause of your pain; they just cover up the symptoms and do damage somewhere else over time in your body.

You Feel That Urge to Have a Pill

The many who suffer know very well that a simple form of movement can make your daily activities difficult with arthritis or any other form of joint pain.

You may feel an urge to have that pain pill to get a quick relief from the inflammation but these anti inflammatory pills have side effects that can lead to permanent damage to the immune system and organs if consumed over time.

Instead of having these pills one should have foods that are anti inflammatory. The foods that are anti inflammatory give a more positive effect to your health.

Here are some foods that are anti inflammatory, healing you faster and having an ongoing effect of healing, and they help in dealing with pain.

Foods That Are Anti Inflammatory

It being said there are thousands of edible plants in the world but humans eat just a small fraction of them. There are plants almost unheard of until recently.

One of the bigger concerns at this point of time is that most don't eat the food they know is good for them, which is crucial for better health. One of the best foods that are anti inflammatory is fish.

Cold water fish such as trout, tuna or salmon are the best because they have loads of anti inflammatory omega 3 fatty acids.

It helps in lowering inflammation. Avoid farmed fish as much as possible. Nuts, like walnuts, almonds, cashews and most others are also rich in omega 3 fatty acids, oleic acid, fibre, protein and phytochemicals which is a very good anti inflammatory food.

When treating inflammation, arthritis and joints, omega is one of the most important nutrient your body needs.

Cold pressed extra Virgin Olive Oil is the healthiest oil for your body, which is a good source of oleic acid and is also known as anti inflammatory oil.

It helps in improving the insulin function, thereby it reduces the blood sugar level. It is however not good for frying because of its low smoke point but it is great for braising and sautéing. Coconut oil for frying is a better option to use.

Cherries: Another excellent food and high in anti inflammatory are the tart cherries, because they are a reach source of antioxidants. It helps in reducing the arthritic inflammation and also reduces the risk of other inflammatory conditions like cancer and cardiovascular diseases.

Leafy Greens: Leafy green vegetables like kale and spinach are also part of the best foods that are anti inflammatory because they are full with antioxidants, omega 3 acids and fibre.

To eliminate possible pesticides and chemicals that may accumulate on the leaves it is necessary to wash them thoroughly.

Green Tea: The unfermented green tea has flavonoids which are known as catechins.

The catechins are the powerful antioxidants which often are destroyed when fermented and processed. The green tea has around 27% of catechins. It helps in reducing inflammation and the symptoms of arthritis.

Apples: Apples contain quercetin which is a chemical with anti inflammatory properties.

Along with other antioxidants it helps in reducing inflammation. The main part of quercetin is present in the skin of the apple; that is why the skin has a red colouring, so it is advisable to not peel off the skin before eating the apple.

Grapes: Grapes have rich anti inflammatory properties as these are high in flavonoids. Drinking pure fresh grape juice without added sugar will also decrease inflammation.

Broccoli: Broccoli, Brussels sprouts and cauliflower help to enhance the immune system and it also helps to combat inflammation.

These contain sulforane that increase the innate detox quality of the body and it also facilitates liver function.

A basic message here is: Eat more food, not more as in quantity, but more in terms of diversity.

The best way of changing your health is the change to a healthy diet.

My name is Josef Bichler I have a passion for wellness and showing others how to live healthy lives.

I have corrected my own health problem with the use of alternatives only and helping others to achieve their health objectives through lifestyle changes exposing unhealthy food to make people aware and understand the benefits of eating healthy and avoiding the culprits that affect our health.

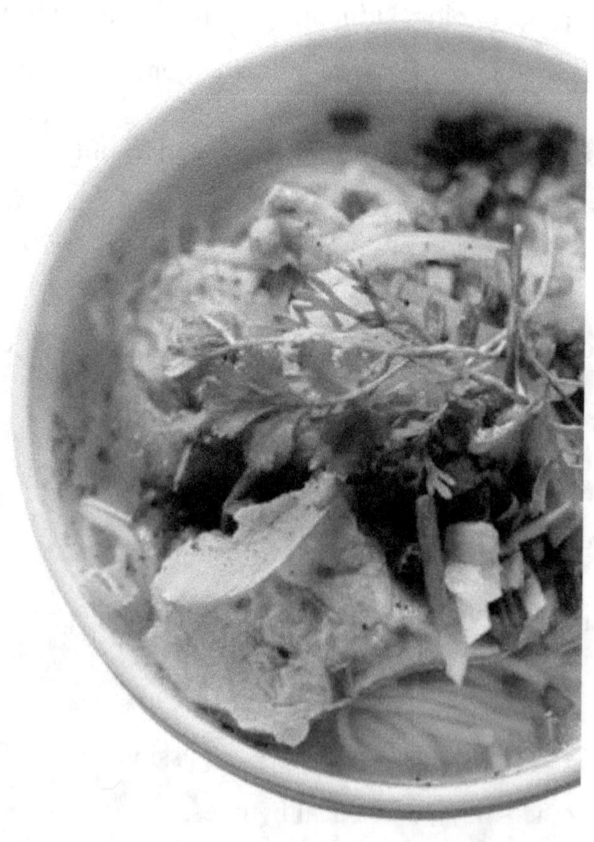

CHAPTER TWO

Top 5 Anti Inflammatory Foods (Best List)

One of the most overlooked causes to some of the most common diseases plaguing our society today is inflammation. Here are the top recommended Anti Inflammatory Foods List and Anti Inflammatory Diet.

When we pour through the statistics, we can see that high blood pressure, asthma, heart disease, and arthritis all have one cause in common and that is inflammation.

The good news is inflammation can be managed simply by making a few changes to your diet. In this article we will look at the most highly recommended anti inflammatory foods and how they can be used to treat and even prevent diseases.

The Essentials. Let's start off by looking at what makes anti inflammatory foods effective and how this can be used to your advantage.

Anti inflammatory foods can mostly be found in an old school diet of fresh fruits and vegetables, with little to no red meat.

Mainly, we are going to look for these three characteristics when considering what foods are a good match:

- An abundance of Omega 3
- High in antioxidants
- Plenty of essential fatty acids.

In essence, this is the Mediterranean diet pioneered by our Greek counterparts. This healing diet features many vegetables, wild fruits, white meat, and seeds with lots of omega 3.

One of the most essential elements to fighting inflammation is maintaining a proper balance between potassium and sodium rich foods.

Both of these minerals work together to clean our body and keep toxins from building up. Now let's look at some of the anti inflammatory diet essentials that we can find at any local grocers.

Bok Choy is one of the most common superfoods.

Bok Choy has recently gained a lot of popularity for its high amount of antioxidants, vitamins, and minerals.Of these, the most notable is something called hydroxycinnamic acids which are powerful antioxidants that will certainly help with inflammation.

Bok Choy is a very robust and versatile vegetable that can go into any veggie dish, making it a staple in the anti inflammatory diet.

Celery and Celery Seeds

The benefits of eating celery are plentiful.

Celery's anti inflammatory abilities have proven to help improve blood pressure, lower cholesterol levels, and even prevent heart disease.

Celery seeds, can be found in many forms, also possess anti inflammatory abilities as well as the added benefit of helping to fight off bacterial infections.

In addition, celery is an excellent healthy source for potassium which our bodies require to flush out toxins.

Blueberries are almost magical in their own right.

A diet rich with blueberries can have many health benefits from improved vision to slower cognitive decline and sharper motor skills.

The antioxidant responsible for blueberry's anti inflammatory benefits is quercetin, which is a substance found in fresh foods that helps to prevent inflammation and even helps to fight cancer.

Benefits don't stop there, one cup of blueberries can contain up to a quarter of your daily source of Vitamins K and C.

Add blueberries to your smoothies or drinks daily.

Salmon is an excellent source of omega 3 and fatty acids.

Several studies have shown that omega 3 fatty acids are essential in lowering the risk of a chronic illness cause by inflammation such as heart disease and arthritis.

In humans, omega 3 is found in the brain and is critical for the health and cognitive function of our brains.

Flaxseeds are one of the most antioxidant packed foods on this list.

Benefits of this wonderful super food include anti aging and improved hormone balance.

Flaxseeds are primarily powered by a phytonutrient called Lignans that provide many antioxidant benefits. To get the most out of this powerful anti inflammatory food, make sure to grind up the seeds. This is so your body can extract the most nutrients.

Anti Inflammatory Food And Fruits To Reduce Joint Pain For Better Results

Joint pain and arthritis can become very uncomfortable and inconveniencing conditions. They can interrupt daily activities, and all the chores we need to do every day. Arthritis inflammation hurts and normal pain killers don't get at the root of the problem. Many people have sought medical attention to ease these conditions and the inflammation related to them. The conditions, largely a result of accumulated toxins, wrong diet and inadequate physical exercise, have an easier way of suppressing them.

Although at an older age it can take longer for inflammation to come back down. Maybe not drugs but some common fruits and change of diet may slow the inflammation pain.

Clinical studies confirmed that natural chemicals in crops can decrease osteoarthritis of the knees and decrease pain in the joints.

The alternative to medical treatment is a comparatively affordable and natural way that will result in a healthy lifestyle at the end of it all.

This involves eating anti inflammatory foods and taking particular interest in anti inflammatory fruits.

Benefits of Anti Inflammatory Fruits

Such fruits are rich in nutrients and minerals that will fight inflammation, just as their name suggests. The fruits particularly contain high quantities of flavonoids, vitamins, and carotenoids. These nutrients, when ingested, will promote action against inflammation and oxidation in the body.

To help you in relieving the pain of inflammation and other health risks, this is what you can do. Alternate these fruits on a daily basis for best results: Blueberries, apples, tart cherries, strawberries, and papaya.

Besides helping you to get rid of inflammation the fruits have other benefits as well.

They will help you lower the risk of cancer and heart disease, will boost your immune system against other diseases, and may help prevent loss of memory.

Daily Diet

You may wonder whether there is a special way that these fruits should be prepared before being eaten.

You can include anti inflammatory fruits, just like any other foods, in the daily diet. Although don't eat fruit straight after the main meal.

Otherwise, just like any other fruit, eat them fresh or direct from the refrigerator, as well as preserved fruits, or make your own juice.

Juices purchased of the shelves are not recommended; that could worsen the situation. Since these fruits have been proven to help joint pain and fight inflammation, it is a good idea to have them included in the family diet for the benefits of every one.

Children, for instance, may not understand the benefits of eating these fruits.

Despite the fruits being very tasty, making them part of meals will make it easy for every family member to boost the immune system.

Having a strong immune system will help your body to defend against illness. Apart from eating the fruits as a main meal, they can also be taken as snacks at any time of the day. They are easy to pick and to eat as you walk away.

Other Anti Inflammatory Foods

Anti inflammatory fruits are not the only natural way to deal with arthritis and inflammation.

There is a wide array of foods to include in the diet such as cold water fish.

Actually, any fish is good because of the omega content which is very important in treating arthritis. Also to include in your diet: Green tea, olive oil, vegetables, turmeric and ginger can offer other options in achieving the same great mission. With this, in a situation where one uses such foods as the main meal, than the anti inflammatory fruits can be eaten in between meals.

Do not use fruit as a dessert after you meal; always eat fruits before a meal for digestion purpose.

However, all of them together will form a formidable force against inflammation.

Whether you are directly affected by this conditions or not, consider anti inflammatory fruits in your diet. If you are free of these conditions, they will help in serving a preventive role.

On the other hand, if you already have arthritis, for instance, they may make that situation better and easier to handle. Keep in mind, the most important step to help any health issue and to a healthier life, is the change to a healthy diet. I have corrected my own health problems with the use of alternatives only and helping others to achieve their health objectives through lifestyle changes, detoxifying their body and through understanding the benefits of selecting foods to fix the problem.

Anti Inflammatory Foods to Add to Your Diet

What does inflammation mean? It is not an infection, although infection can cause inflammation.

Actually inflammation is the body's own defence attempt to remove harmful stimuli, such as irritants, damaged cells etc. This is when inflammation is trying its healing process.

Inflammation is the first sign when something harmful or irritating is affecting parts of our body. Every one's body has an immune system and inflammation is part of that. Inflammation is also a localized physical condition that results as a reaction to an injury or infection, causing parts of the body to become swollen, reddened, painful and hot. Internal inflammation can happen due to eating of processed foods, fats and sugars.

High levels of inflammation can cause a number of health complications such as arthritis, joint pain, damage to blood vessels among others. To combat this, it is important you eat foods that are anti inflammatory. Such foods are readily available to add to your diet to curb inflammation. Here are some of the foods and suggestions to help and keep harmful inflammation at bay:

Whole Grains

When it comes to whole grains it is better you consume your grains as whole grains and not refined or pasta.

Research has shown that whole grains contain a high amount of fibre which reduces the inflammatory marker in blood known as C reactive protein.

Dark Leafy Greens

Dark leafy vegetables such as spinach and kale have high concentrations of vitamin E and minerals such as calcium and iron.

Studies show that vitamin E helps in protecting your body from inflammatory molecules known as cytokines. Additionally, dark leafy greens have a high amount of disease fighting phytochemicals.

Fatty Fish

Oily fish such as salmon and tuna are foods that are anti inflammatory as they contain high amounts of omega 3 fatty acids.

The fatty acids are known to help joint inflammation, so make sure you get plenty of omega 3. Another important fact about omega 3 is you must get it in your food because the body cannot make it within its system.

Soy

Soybeans contain isoflavones compounds which help the negative effects of inflammation on joints.

However, it is good you avoid heavily processed soy products as they may contain additives and preservatives. Instead, include soy milk and soy beans into your regular diet.

Nuts

Nuts such as almonds and walnuts are rich in vitamin E, calcium and fibre.

All nuts are full of antioxidants which can help the body in repairing the damages caused by inflammation.

Berries

Berries are low in fat and calories but rich in antioxidants.

Their anti inflammatory anthocyanins compound in them has many good qualities. This helps to prevent you from developing arthritis.

Green Tea

Green tea as well has anti inflammatory flavonoids; this reduces the onset of inflammation and minimizes the risk of certain cancers.

It shouldn't be underestimated for many other health benefits. It can reactivate skin cells making skin appear brighter. Drink it regularly and use some honey as a sweetener instead of sugar.

Low Fat Dairy

Low fat dairy such as yogurt contains probiotics which can prevent inflammation. Additionally, dairy foods that are anti inflammatory such as skim milk with high calcium and vitamin D are important for everyone since apart from having anti inflammatory properties, they strengthen your bones also.

Ginger and Garlic

Ginger and garlic are foods that are anti inflammatory. Both are known to lower body inflammation, control blood sugar levels and help your body in fighting certain infections. Selenium and sulphur in garlic is an essential compound for a healthy immune system. It is also one of the top anti aging foods you can eat.

Turmeric and Sweet Potato

Turmeric has natural anti inflammatory compounds called curcumin which is known to turn off NF kappa B protein that triggers the process of inflammation. On the other hand, sweet potato is a good source of fibre, vitamin B 6, vitamin C, complex carbohydrates and better carotene. These ingredients help to heal inflammation in your body. These are some of many foods that are anti inflammatory which can help you in reducing joint pain and arthritis caused by inflammation. Add them to your diet.

However, reduce foods that are high in fats especially trans fats and sugar as they can spur inflammation, joint pain, arthritis, and damage blood vessels among other related inflammatory conditions. Making a few changes will improve many things and can have you feeling more energetic and alive than you have in a long time, and will continue to do so as long as you stay with the changes you made. This is where many go wrong.

When things have improved they go back to the same old way as before. Don't sabotage your own health; stick with what you are doing, the changes you made, that made you feel better.

Don't go back to the old ways what you've done before.

My name is Josef Bichler I have a passion for wellness and showing others how to live healthy lives. I have corrected my own health problems with the use of alternatives only.

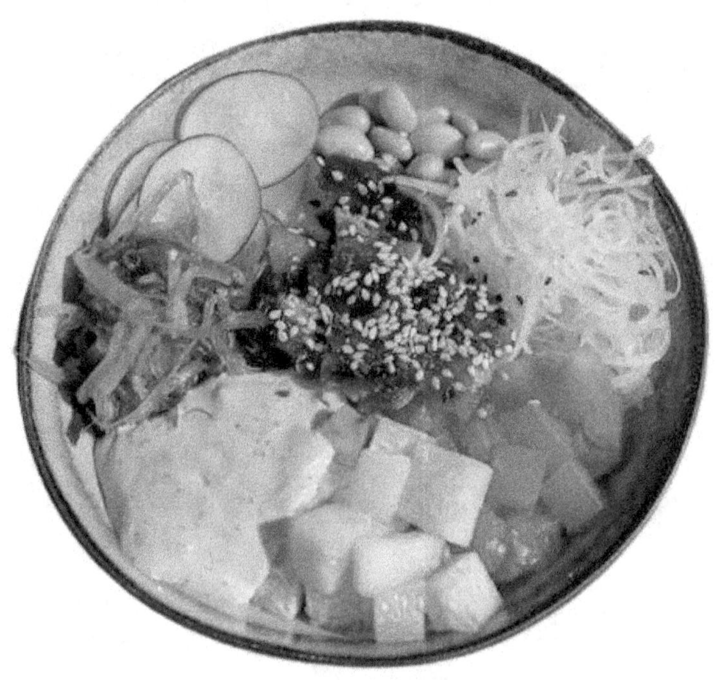

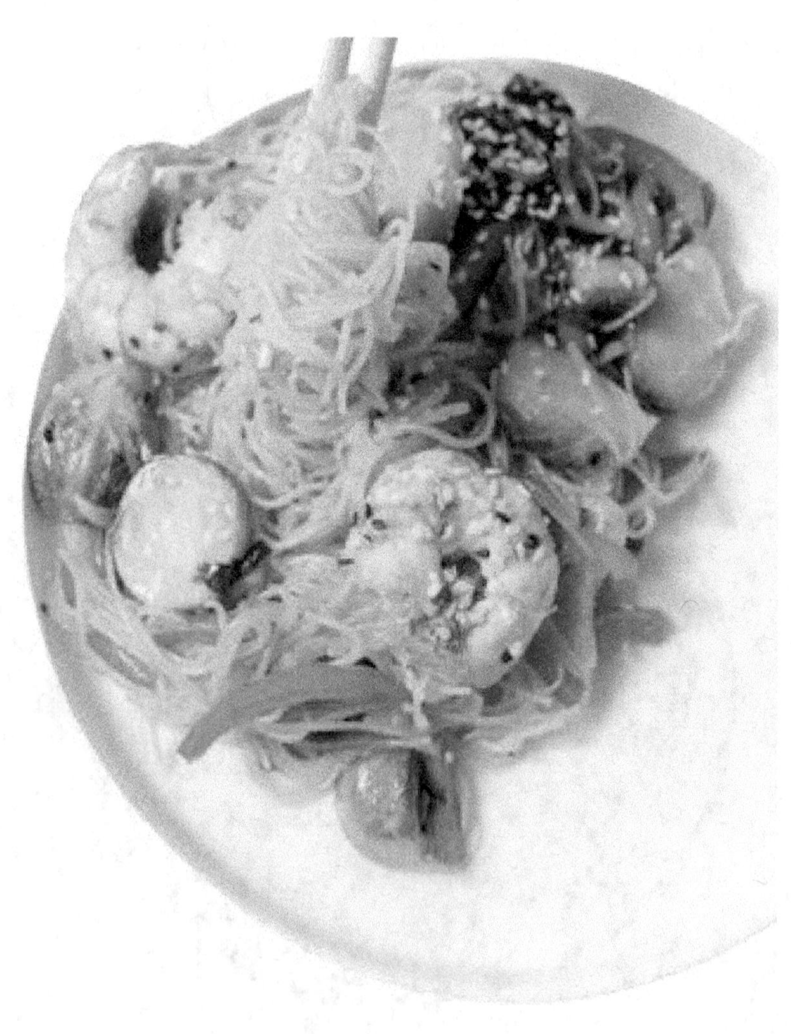

CHAPTER THREE

Anti Inflammatory Foods How Important Are They In Our Life?

What are anti inflammatory foods? They are foods that reduce swelling in the body, promote better health and many more things. They are far important that we can realize.

Inflammation is distinct as a restricted response of tissue to injury, irritation, or infection.

There are symptoms such as pain, swelling, loss of movement, and redness to the area. Although most people imagine it as being chronic arthritis, or painful muscles, but the medical profession are now looking at heart malady and strokes being linked to it as well.

By having natural anti inflammatory foods on your diet, it is felt that you can now stop the pain and stave off serious illness.

Inflammation is part of your body's defense system against harmful bacteria and viruses, but scientists now believe that when it remains, it can cause a lot of problems.

Make sure you take care of yourself by leading a healthy lifestyle. You should take regular exercise, stop smoking, try to reduce the stress of everyday life, and try to maintain your weight at an acceptable level.

This will help to reduce inflammation, but the best way is to change your eating habits.

Adding anti inflammatory foods and supplements to your diet will greatly reduce the possibilities of chronic illness. Cut down on fatty sources such as red meat, and processed convenience foods.

To counter inflammation, we should be eating lots of fruit and vegetables. Fish is also good, though now there is the suggestion that some fish are polluted and contain high levels of mercury, and other toxins.

The smaller fish, such as sardines and anchovies are considered to be healthy, and fish oil supplements are also recommended.

Whether or not you can gain those benefits from anti inflammatory foods it depends on your willingness to start an eating plan based on them and to enjoy what you do.

Basically, most dieting is common sense, and the motivation to live a healthy lifestyle.

Anti Inflammatory Diet: What To Know

Inflammation helps the body fight illness and can protect it from harm. In most cases, it is a necessary part of the healing process.

However, some people have a medical condition in which the immune system does not work as it should. This malfunction can lead to persistent or recurrent low level inflammation.

Chronic inflammation occurs with various diseases, such as psoriasis, rheumatoid arthritis, and asthma.

There is evidence that dietary choices may help manage the symptoms.

An anti inflammatory diet favors fruits and vegetables, foods containing omega 3 fatty acids, whole grains, lean protein, healthful fats, and spices. It discourages or limits the consumption of processed foods, red meats, and alcohol. The anti inflammatory diet is not a specific regimen but rather a style of eating. The Mediterranean diet and the DASH diet are examples of anti inflammatory diets.

What is an anti inflammatory diet?

Some foods contain ingredients that can trigger or worsen inflammation. Sugary or processed foods may do this, while fresh, whole foods are less likely to have this effect.

An anti inflammatory diet focuses on fresh fruits and vegetables. Many plant based foods are good sources of antioxidants.

Some foods, however, can triggerTrusted Source the formation of free radicals. Examples include foods that people fry in repeatedly heated cooking oil.

Dietary molecules in food that help remove free radicals from the body.

Free radicals are the natural byproducts of some bodily processes, including metabolism. However, external factors, such as stress and smoking, can increase the number of free radicals in the body.

Free radicals can lead to cell damage. This damage increases the risk of inflammation and can contribute to a range of diseases.

The body creates some antioxidants that help it remove these toxic substances, but dietary antioxidants also help.

An anti inflammatory diet favors foods that are rich in antioxidants over those that increase the production of free radicals.

Omega 3 fatty acids, which are present in oily fish, may help reduce the levels of inflammatory proteins in the body. Fiber can also have this effect, according to the Arthritis Foundation.

Which foods are good sources of antioxidants? Find out here.

Types of anti inflammatory diet

Many popular diets already adhere to anti inflammatory principles.

For example, both the Mediterranean diet and the DASH diet include fresh fruits and vegetables, fish, whole grains, and fats that are good for the heart.

Inflammation appears to play a role in cardiovascular disease, but researchTrusted Source suggests that the Mediterranean diet, with its focus on plant based foods and healthful oils, can reduce the effects of inflammation on the cardiovascular system.

Who can it help?

An anti inflammatory diet may serve as a complementary therapy for many conditions that become worse with chronic inflammation.

The following conditions involve inflammation:

Rheumatoid arthritis, Psoriasis, Asthma, Eosinophilic esophagitis, Crohn's disease, Colitis, Inflammatory bowel disease, Lupus, Hashimoto's thyroiditis, Metabolic syndrome

Foods to eat

- Tuna and salmon
- Fruits, such as blueberries, blackberries, strawberries, and cherries
- Vegetables, including kale, spinach, and broccoli
- Beans, Nuts and seeds, Olives and olive oil and Fiber.

Also recommended:

- Raw or moderately cooked vegetables
- Legumes, such as lentils
- Spices, such as ginger and turmeric

- Probiotics and prebiotics

- Tea

- Some herbs.

It is worth remembering that:

No single food will boost a person's health. It is important to include a variety of healthful ingredients in the diet.

Fresh, simple ingredients are best. Processing can change the nutritional content of foods.

People should check the labels of premade foods. While cocoa can be a good choice, for example, the products that contain cocoa often also contain sugar and fat.

A colorful plate will provide a range of antioxidants and other nutrients.

Be sure to vary the colors of fruits and vegetables.

Foods to avoid

People who are following an anti inflammatory diet should avoid or limit their intake of:

- Processed foods

- Foods with added sugar or salt

- Unhealthful oils

- processed carbs, which are present in white bread, white pasta, and many baked goods

- Processed snack foods, such as chips and crackers

- Premade desserts, such as cookies, candy, and ice cream

- Excess alcohol.

In addition, people may find it beneficial to limit their intake of the following:

Gluten: Some people experience an inflammatory reaction when they consume gluten. A gluten free diet can be restrictive, and it is not suitable for everyone.

However, if a person suspects that gluten is triggering symptoms, they may wish to consider eliminating it for a while to see if their symptoms improve.

Nightshades: Plants belonging to the nightshade family, such as tomatoes, eggplants, peppers, and potatoes, seem to trigger flares in some people with inflammatory diseases.

There is limited evidence to confirm this effect, but a person can try cutting nightshades from the diet for 2–3 weeks to see if their symptoms improve.

Carbohydrates: There is some evidence that a high carb diet, even when the carbs are healthful, may promote inflammation in some people.

However, some carb rich foods, such as sweet potatoes and whole grains, are excellent sources of antioxidants and other nutrients.

Who Needs an Anti Inflammatory Diet?

Inflammation is often associated with injury. You stub your toe and the toe swells.

This is the basic inflammatory reaction. Some people even understand that redness around a cut is also a form of inflammation that the immune system uses to heal the injury.

What is not commonly known is the fact that inflammation occurs inside the body as well. When the body exists in an inflammatory state, risk of illness, cancer and heart conditions can increase. An anti inflammatory diet is an easy way to combat this aftereffect and reduce risk today.

I don't suffer from Inflammation!

This is the most common statement and the least correct.

Inflammation affects every person in the world at some point in their life. In western cultures, like the United States, a huge portion of the population is affected by inflammation every day. Being overweight or obese is the most common inflammatory condition. It is this inflammatory response that could be the cause of some weight related conditions like diabetes.

When fat cells grow, they take up the free space around the organs.

Blood flow can be constricted and the body often feels as though it needs to fight to function normally. When the body feels threatened, inflammation occurs as a natural, healing response.

Unfortunately, unlike the small cut that will heal in a few, short days. Obesity takes time to correct and the longer the body lives inflamed, the greater the risk of long term effects.

In the case of obesity, changing the diet by reducing calories will reduce body weight and thus reduce the inflammation in the body.

This is the simplest benefit of an anti inflammatory diet. However, people who are obese or overweight are not the only people who can benefit from an anti inflammatory diet.

Illness Treatment and Prevention

There are many illnesses and conditions caused by inflammation.

These include asthma, arthritis, inflammatory bowel syndrome, pelvic inflammatory disease, endometriosis, diabetes, COPD, Psoriasis, Colitis, and Lupus just to name a few. All in all, there are nearly 40 autoimmune conditions currently accepted by the medical community that are affected by inflammation.

What Can I Do?

The first step is to make dietary changes to reduce food based inflammation. Processed foods, fast foods and prepackaged foods can cause increased inflammation in the body.

Replacing these foods with lean meats, whole grains and healthy fats will make a tremendous different in how the body reacts to inflammation.

In addition, if weight is a problem, reducing weight while changing to an anti inflammatory diet can increase the benefits exponentially.

Changing to an anti inflammatory diet does not have to be in reaction to a disease or illness.

Prevention is the best choice and the anti inflammatory diet can reduce the risk of contracting many of the listed illnesses.

When the body feels as though it needs to fight for survival, inflammation occurs, so offering healthy foods that have an inflammatory effect is a great choice for all people including those who are young, healthy and feel they do not need an anti inflammatory diet.

CHAPTER FOUR

Other Health Benefits of An Anti Inflammatory Diet

While each plan has its own twist, all are based on the general concept that constant or out of control inflammation in the body leads to ill health, and that eating to avoid constant inflammation promotes better health and can ward off disease, says Russell Greenfield, MD, a clinical assistant professor of medicine at the University of North Carolina at Chapel Hill and a private practice physician who studied under Weil.

It's very clear that inflammation plays a role much more than we thought with respect to certain maladies.

We always thought anything with an ' it is' at the end involved inflammation," he says, such as arthritis or appendicitis. But even the illnesses without an it is at the end, such as cardiovascular disease, certain cancers, even Alzheimer's disease, may be triggered in part by inflammation.

Sears calls inflammation a silent epidemic that triggers chronic diseases over the years. "You could feel fine but have high levels of inflammation," he warns.

The average American diet, Greenfield says, includes far too many foods rich in omega 6 fatty acids, found in processed and fast foods, and far too few rich in omega 3 fatty acids, such as those found in cold water fish or supplements.

 When that balance is out of whack, inflammation can set in, Sears explains.

Phytochemicals   natural chemicals found in the plant foods suggested on the diets   are also believed to help reduce inflammation.

Anti Inflammatory Diets: What Do You Eat?

An exact description of the anti inflammatory diet varies, depending on whom you ask. The anti inflammatory diet is "probably very close to the Mediterranean diet," says Christopher Cannon, MD, associate professor of medicine at Harvard Medical School and a cardiologist at Brigham and Women's Hospital, Boston.

He co authored "The Complete Idiot's Guide to The Anti Inflammation Diet," which includes recipes for anti inflammatory eating and information on vitamins.

An anti inflammatory diet is the Zone diet with fish oil, says Sears, who wrote "The Anti Inflammation Zone" and whose popular Zone diet recommends low fat protein, carbs, and heart healthy monounsaturated fats.

Specifics vary from diet to diet, but in general anti inflammatory diets suggest:

- Eat plenty of fruits and vegetables.
- Minimize saturated and trans fats.
- Eat a good source of omega 3 fatty acids, such as fish or fish oil supplements and walnuts.
- Watch your intake of refined carbohydrates such as pasta and white rice.
- Eat plenty of whole grains such as brown rice and bulgur wheat.
- Eat lean protein sources such as chicken; cut back on red meat and full fat dairy foods.
- Avoid refined foods and processed foods.

    – Spice it up. Ginger, curry, and other spices can have an anti inflammatory effect.

As one example of a day's worth of anti inflammatory eating, Cannon suggests a breakfast of toasted steel cut oatmeal with berries, yogurt, or other topping and coffee or green tea.

Lunch could be tuna salad on 7 grain bread and a smoothie with seasonal fruits.

For a snack, try an ounce of dark chocolate and about four walnuts. Dinner could be spaghetti with turkey meat sauce, spinach salad with oranges and walnuts, and apple cranberry pie made without butter.

The diets don't promise weight loss, but weight reduction does often occur. And that makes sense, given the makeup of the diet.

When you are talking about cutting back on red meat, dairy, fats and trans fats, partially hydrogenated oils, highly processed carbs and eating healthier protein like fish, eating more fruits and vegetables   odds are that people are going to lose at least a little bit of weight.

Proponents say it can, but they acknowledge that the anti inflammatory diet needs to be studied more extensively to prove that it actually reduces disease such as heart problems.

But a related diet, the Mediterranean diet, has been and is associated with improved cardiac outcomes.

There is ample evidence [of disease risk reduction] on the Asian style diet and the Mediterranean style diet. When you take a look at the components [of those diets], they could easily be called anti inflammatory diets.

And eating a diet high in omega 6 and low in omega 3 is associated with increasing levels of cytokines   proteins released from cells that trigger inflammation   according to a study published in Psychosomatic Medicine.

Omega 3, in doses of 3 grams or more per day, has been found effective for those with rheumatoid arthritis, reducing morning stiffness and the number of joints that are tender or swollen, according to a review of the research on omega 3 fatty acids and health in American Family Physician.

Anecdotally, says Greenfield, he hears from patients that avoiding "inflammatory" foods can help their osteoarthritis pain.

He recalls talking to patients with arthritis who have vacationed in India, for instance, eating dishes with plenty of curry, and telling him their joints didn't hurt as much while they were there.

Curry, he says, as well as ginger, is a natural anti inflammatory.

Not surprisingly, the anti inflammatory diet takes longer to work than, say, an anti inflammatory medicine. "With an anti inflammatory drug, you feel better in an hour or two," Greenfield says.

For the anti inflammatory diet, more patience is needed. "I would say clearly within just a few weeks most of the patients I have see a noticeable difference [in symptoms]."

Anti Inflammatory Diets: More Opinions

It's not surprising that anti inflammatory diets have gotten popular, says Elisa Zied, RD, a spokeswoman for the American Dietetic Association and a dietitian in New York City.

While they may have some merit, she cautions: "Individual foods should not be the focus. You need to pay attention to your overall pattern." And reducing inflammation is not just about what you eat, she says.

"Maintaining a healthy body weight is the best thing you can do to reduce inflammation," Zied says.

Patience White, MD, the chief public health officer for the Arthritis Foundation, agrees, particularly when it comes to patients with arthritis.

"The link between weight and osteoarthritis in the lower extremities is very close," she says. "The heavier you are, the more likely you are to get arthritis.

12 Easy Ways To Reduce Inflammation Overnight

Here's how to tamp down inflammation and reduce your chronic disease risk in as little as one day.

The subject of inflammation is everywhere lately, and the hype is for good reason. Not only can adopting an anti inflammatory diet and lifestyle reduce chronic inflammation to help you stay healthy and slow down aging, but research also suggests it can reduce your risk of heart disease, diabetes, dementia, Alzheimer's disease, autoimmune diseases, joint pain, and cancer.

Best part? You don't have to wait for months or years to start seeing results and feeling better! Small changes you make today can start reducing your inflammation overnight. Here's what to do ASAP to start reaping the health benefits.

1. Eat a salad every day

Keep a package or two of leafy greens on hand to toss in your lunch bag or on your dinner plate.

Having a cup of leafy greens—like baby spinach, arugula, kale, or lettuce—each day is one of the most beneficial diet habits you can adopt.

These leafy greens offer an anti inflammatory double punch, thanks to antioxidants and bioactive compounds that reduce inflammation and prevent free radicals from creating new inflammation.

2. Avoid getting angry

Skip the vending machine and sweetened coffee drinks, and opt instead for a fiber rich snack with a little protein like apple slices and peanut butter, raw veggies and hummus, or a few almonds and cheese cubes.

The reason is that eating a balanced snack without added sugars and refined carbs is key to keeping blood sugar within normal parameters, which in turn helps you avoid cravings, hunger, and irritability.

Not only is this nicer for those around you, but avoiding peaks and drops in blood sugar also prevents inflammation in the body that can lead to obesity, Type 2 diabetes, and heart disease.

3. Go to bed

Turn off Netflix, get off social media, and head to bed a little earlier. While it may seem a little indulgent, getting 7 to 8 hours of continuous sleep is what's considered adequate for adults and we should all aim for that as our norm.

Routinely not getting enough sleep (6 hours or less) triggers inflammation—even in healthy individuals—which research suggests increases risk for metabolic issues that can lead to obesity, Type 2 diabetes, and heart disease, as well as dementia and Alzheimer's.

4. Take your dog for a walk

Missed your workout today? Take a quick walk around the block!

While regular exercise is ideal for treating and preventing most all health issues, some days there's not enough time for a full blown workout.

However, results from a 2017 study suggest that getting just 20 minutes of movement reduces inflammatory blood markers. So, lace up your shoes and get going!

5. Spice things up

Look for ways to add a little garlic or spice when you're cooking dinner tonight.

Fragrant and pungent spices seem like they would have the potential to aggravate inflammation, but research suggests they actually do the opposite.

In fact, there's evidence to suggest incorporating garlic, or herbs and spices such as turmeric, rosemary, cinnamon, cumin, ginger, and fenugreek, decreases inflammation that could eventually lead to heart disease, brain degenerative conditions, cancer, and respiratory issues.

6. Take a break from alcohol

If you like having a nightly cocktail or glass of wine, consider abstaining for a few days.

This doesn't have to be long term, but cutting out alcohol briefly (while making other anti inflammatory diet and lifestyle changes) helps the body calm down and reduce existing inflammation.

While research suggests that moderate alcohol consumption offers some benefits, the problem is that it's easy to cross the line from beneficial and anti inflammatory to harmful and inflammatory.

7. Swap one coffee for green tea

If you drink 1 to 3 cups of coffee or other caffeinated drinks a day, consider swapping one of those for a cup of green tea instead.

Green tea leaves are packed with polyphenol compounds, which can help reduce free radical damage to stop further inflammation. Studies suggest that regularly drinking green tea can help reduce your risk of Alzheimer's disease, cancer, and joint conditions.

8. Be gentle to your gut

There's lots of hype around probiotics, but are you supporting those good microbes already living in you?

Protect those existing good bacteria by cutting out added sugars, trans fats, and focusing on choosing primarily whole and minimally processed foods.

It's also worth consuming probiotic rich foods—such as yogurt, sauerkraut, kombucha, miso, or kimchi—every single day.

Strengthening the gut's microbe barrier is one of the cornerstones to reducing inflammation long term.

9. Consider a fast

Granted, it's not for everyone, but research continues to find benefits when it comes to intermittent fasting (IF), largely due to the anti inflammatory effects the eating pattern induces.

There are several ways to approach fasting, but an easy way to start is with a 12 hour fast.

This means if you finish dinner at 7 p.m., then you only consume water or black coffee until 7 a.m. the next day.

Studies suggest regularly doing IF may reduce heart disease risk and improve insulin sensitivity, brain health, and inflammatory bowel disease.

10. Cut out dairy and gluten (temporarily)

Dairy and gluten are not usually inflammatory in healthy individuals (unless you have an allergy, intolerance, or celiac disease), but they can be irritating when there's already existing inflammation. Some people may find it beneficial to cut out dairy, gluten, or both for a few weeks while eating a diet rich in anti inflammatory foods and low in inflammatory ones.

The thought is that this gives the body time to "calm down." After which, you can slowly start to incorporate dairy or gluten containing foods to see if they cause any irritation.

11. Chill out

No matter how healthy your diet, low grade inflammation isn't going away if stress levels run continuously high. And even if stress isn't too much of daily problem, learning how to manage and cope when it does occur is key for preventing new inflammation.

Finding healthy ways to escape that stress—for example, by practicing yoga, meditating, or taking a short walk—provides quick relief psychologically and anti inflammatory effects physiologically.

12. Be picky about ingredients

Additives, dyes, preservatives, and other ingredients regularly added to foods all have the potential to trigger or aggravate inflammation—particularly if you have a weaker gut barrier—so take a look at the ingredient list on products in your pantry and fridge.

Are the ingredients listed what you might use if making the food from a recipe at home? If yes, then this is likely a minimally processed product and a good choice.

 If not, opt for another brand or substitute when shopping next time.

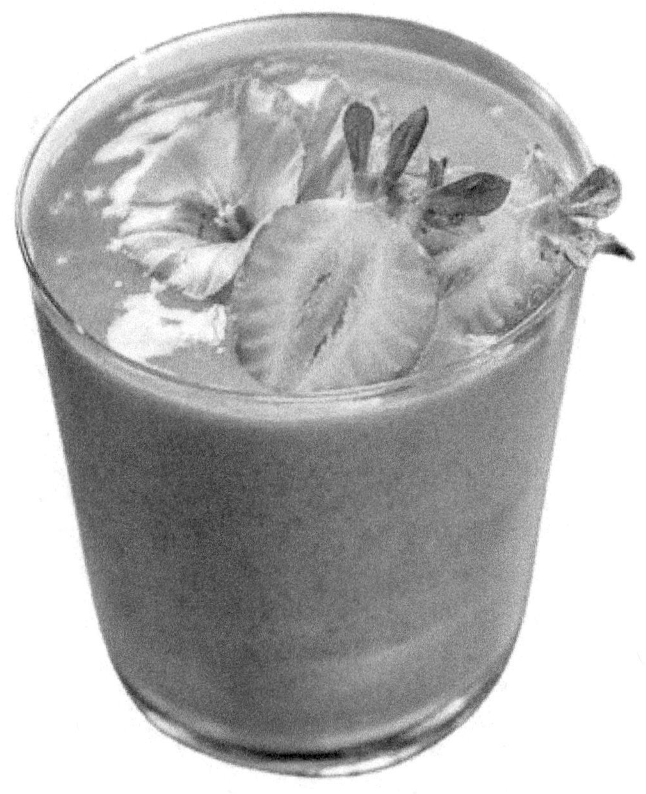

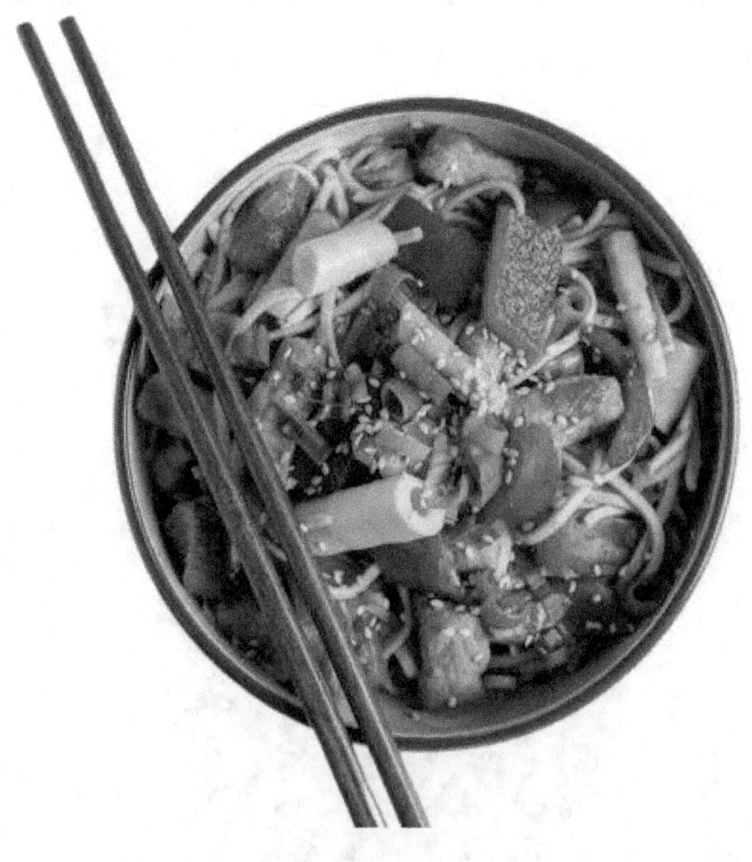

CHAPTER FIVE

Anti Inflammatory Meal Prep Recipes

1. Turmeric Chickpea Quinoa Bowl

Ingredients:

- 1 cup cooked quinoa
- 1 can (15 oz) chickpeas, drained and rinsed
- 1 teaspoon turmeric powder
- 1/2 teaspoon ground cumin
- 1/2 teaspoon ground coriander
- 1 tablespoon olive oil
- 2 cups mixed greens
- 1/4 cup diced cucumber
- 1/4 cup diced red bell pepper
- Lemon tahini dressing (lemon juice, tahini, and water mixed to desired consistency)
- Salt and pepper to taste

Method:

1. In a bowl, mix chickpeas with turmeric, cumin, coriander, olive oil, salt, and pepper.
2. Spread chickpeas on a baking sheet and roast at 375°F (190°C) for 20 minutes until crispy.
3. Divide quinoa, roasted chickpeas, mixed greens, cucumber, and red bell pepper into meal prep containers.
4. Drizzle each container with lemon tahini dressing before serving.

2. Salmon and Asparagus Sheet Pan Meal

Ingredients:

- 4 salmon fillets
- 1 bunch asparagus, trimmed
- 2 tablespoons olive oil
- 1 teaspoon garlic powder
- 1 teaspoon lemon zest
- Salt and pepper to taste
- Fresh dill for garnish

Method:

1. Preheat your oven to 425°F (220°C).

2. Place salmon fillets and asparagus on a baking sheet.

3. Drizzle with olive oil and season with garlic powder, lemon zest, salt, and pepper.

4. Bake for 15 20 minutes until salmon flakes easily with a fork.

5. Divide into meal prep containers, garnish with fresh dill, and store.

3. Anti Inflammatory Green Smoothie

Ingredients:

-   1 cup kale or spinach
-   1/2 cup pineapple chunks
-   1/2 inch piece of fresh ginger, peeled
-   1/2 teaspoon turmeric powder
-   1 tablespoon chia seeds
-   1 cup unsweetened almond milk
-   Ice cubes (optional)

Method:

1. Blend kale/spinach, pineapple, ginger, turmeric, chia seeds, and almond milk until smooth.
2. Add ice cubes if desired and blend again.
3. Pour into individual jars or bottles for a quick and nutritious breakfast or snack.

4. Mediterranean Chickpea Salad

Ingredients:

- 2 cups cooked chickpeas
- 1 cucumber, diced
- 1 cup cherry tomatoes, halved
- 1/4 cup red onion, finely chopped
- 1/4 cup fresh parsley, chopped
- 2 tablespoons extra virgin olive oil
- Juice of 1 lemon
- 1 teaspoon dried oregano
- Salt and pepper to taste

Method:

1. In a large bowl, combine chickpeas, cucumber, cherry tomatoes, red onion, and parsley.
2. Whisk together olive oil, lemon juice, oregano, salt, and pepper to make the dressing.
3. Pour the dressing over the salad and toss well.
4. Divide into meal prep containers and refrigerate.

5. Roasted Vegetable and Quinoa Bowl

Ingredients:

- 2 cups cooked quinoa
- 1 cup broccoli florets
- 1 cup cauliflower florets
- 1 cup sweet potato cubes
- 2 tablespoons olive oil
- 1 teaspoon smoked paprika
- 1/2 teaspoon ground turmeric
- Salt and pepper to taste
- Tahini sauce (tahini, lemon juice, water, and garlic)

Method:

1. Preheat your oven to 425°F (220°C).
2. Toss broccoli, cauliflower, and sweet potato with olive oil, smoked paprika, turmeric, salt, and pepper.
3. Roast for 20 25 minutes until veggies are tender.
4. Divide quinoa and roasted veggies into meal prep containers.
5. Drizzle with tahini sauce before serving.

6. Spinach and Quinoa Stuffed Bell Peppers

Ingredients:

- 4 bell peppers, halved and cleaned
- 1 cup cooked quinoa
- 1 cup fresh spinach, chopped
- 1 can (15 oz) black beans, drained and rinsed
- 1/2 cup diced tomatoes
- 1 teaspoon ground cumin
- 1/2 teaspoon smoked paprika
- Salt and pepper to taste
- 1/4 cup shredded cheese (optional)

Method:

1. Preheat your oven to 375°F (190°C).
2. In a bowl, mix cooked quinoa, chopped spinach, black beans, diced tomatoes, ground cumin, smoked paprika, salt, and pepper.
3. Fill each bell pepper half with the quinoa mixture.
4. Place stuffed bell peppers in a baking dish and cover with aluminum foil.
5. Bake for 25 30 minutes, remove the foil, and continue baking for an additional 10 minutes until peppers are tender.
6. Optionally, sprinkle shredded cheese on top before serving.

7. Berry and Walnut Overnight Oats

Ingredients:

- 1 cup rolled oats
- 1 cup unsweetened almond milk
- 1/2 cup mixed berries (blueberries, strawberries, raspberries)
- 1/4 cup chopped walnuts

- 1 tablespoon honey or maple syrup

- 1/2 teaspoon ground cinnamon

Method:

1. In a mason jar or container, layer rolled oats, mixed berries, and chopped walnuts.
2. Drizzle honey or maple syrup over the layers and sprinkle with ground cinnamon.
3. Pour almond milk over the top and seal the jar/container.
4. Refrigerate overnight, and your breakfast is ready to go.

8. Roasted Garlic and Lemon Broccoli

Ingredients:

- 2 cups broccoli florets

- 2 cloves garlic, minced

- Zest and juice of 1 lemon

- 1 tablespoon olive oil

- Salt and pepper to taste

Method:

1. Preheat your oven to 425°F (220°C).

2. Toss broccoli florets with minced garlic, lemon zest, lemon juice, olive oil, salt, and pepper.

3. Spread the mixture on a baking sheet and roast for 15 20 minutes until broccoli is tender and slightly crispy.

4. Divide into meal prep containers for a flavorful side dish.

9. Cilantro Lime Shrimp Bowl

Ingredients:

- 8 oz cooked shrimp

- 1 cup cooked brown rice

- 1/2 cup black beans, drained and rinsed

- 1/2 cup diced red bell pepper

- 1/4 cup fresh cilantro, chopped

- Juice of 1 lime

- 1 tablespoon olive oil

- Salt and pepper to taste

- Sliced avocado for garnish (optional)

Method:

1. In a bowl, combine cooked shrimp, brown rice, black beans, diced red bell pepper, and fresh cilantro.
2. In a separate small bowl, whisk together lime juice, olive oil, salt, and pepper to create the dressing.
3. Pour the dressing over the shrimp and rice mixture and toss well.
4. Garnish with sliced avocado before serving.

10. Berry Spinach Salad with Almond Dressing

Ingredients:

- 2 cups baby spinach
- 1/2 cup mixed berries (strawberries, blueberries, raspberries)
- 1/4 cup sliced almonds
- 1/4 cup red onion, thinly sliced
- Almond dressing (blend almonds, water, lemon juice, and a touch of honey)

Method:

1. In a bowl, combine baby spinach, mixed berries, sliced almonds, and red onion.

2. Drizzle the almond dressing over the salad before serving.

11. Baked Salmon with Dill and Turmeric

Ingredients:

- 4 salmon fillets
- 1 tablespoon olive oil
- 1 teaspoon dried dill
- 1/2 teaspoon ground turmeric
- Salt and pepper to taste
- Lemon wedges for garnish

Method:

1. Preheat your oven to 375°F (190°C).

2. Place salmon fillets on a baking sheet.

3. Drizzle olive oil over the salmon and season with dried dill, ground turmeric, salt, and pepper.

4. Bake for 15 20 minutes or until the salmon flakes easily with a fork.

5. Divide into meal prep containers and garnish with lemon wedges.

12. Quinoa and Lentil Salad

Ingredients:

- 1 cup cooked quinoa
- 1 cup cooked green or brown lentils
- 1 cup diced cucumber
- 1 cup cherry tomatoes, halved
- 1/4 cup red onion, finely chopped
- 2 tablespoons fresh mint leaves, chopped
- 2 tablespoons extra virgin olive oil
- Juice of 1 lemon
- Salt and pepper to taste

Method:

1. In a bowl, combine quinoa, cooked lentils, cucumber, cherry tomatoes, red onion, and fresh mint.
2. In a separate small bowl, whisk together olive oil, lemon juice, salt, and pepper to make the dressing.
3. Drizzle the dressing over the salad and toss well.
4. Portion into meal prep containers and refrigerate.

13. Spiced Sweet Potato Soup

Ingredients:

- 2 cups sweet potatoes, peeled and diced
- 1 cup carrots, peeled and chopped
- 1 onion, chopped
- 2 cloves garlic, minced
- 1 teaspoon ground turmeric
- 1/2 teaspoon ground ginger
- 4 cups vegetable broth
- 1 tablespoon olive oil
- Salt and pepper to taste
- Fresh cilantro for garnish

Method:

1. Heat olive oil in a large pot over medium heat.

2. Add chopped onion and garlic, sauté until fragrant.

3. Add diced sweet potatoes, carrots, ground turmeric, and ground ginger. Sauté for a few more minutes.

4. Pour in vegetable broth, bring to a boil, then reduce heat and simmer until the vegetables are tender (about 20 25 minutes).

5. Use an immersion blender to blend the soup until smooth.

6. Season with salt and pepper, garnish with fresh cilantro, and portion into meal prep containers.

14. Greek Quinoa Salad

Ingredients:

- 1 cup cooked quinoa
- 1/2 cup diced cucumber
- 1/2 cup cherry tomatoes, halved
- 1/4 cup Kalamata olives, pitted and sliced
- 1/4 cup crumbled feta cheese
- 2 tablespoons extra virgin olive oil
- Juice of 1 lemon

- 1 teaspoon dried oregano
- Salt and pepper to taste

Method:

1. In a bowl, combine cooked quinoa, diced cucumber, cherry tomatoes, Kalamata olives, and crumbled feta cheese.
2. In a separate small bowl, whisk together olive oil, lemon juice, dried oregano, salt, and pepper to create the dressing.
3. Drizzle the dressing over the salad and toss well.
4. Divide into meal prep containers and refrigerate.

15. Almond and Blueberry Protein Bars

Ingredients:

- 1 cup almonds
- 1 cup dried blueberries
- 1/4 cup honey or maple syrup
- 1/4 cup almond butter
- 1/4 cup unsweetened protein powder
- 1/2 teaspoon ground cinnamon

Method:

1. In a food processor, combine almonds, dried blueberries, honey or maple syrup, almond butter, protein powder, and ground cinnamon.
2. Process until the mixture comes together and forms a sticky dough.
3. Press the mixture into a lined baking pan and refrigerate for at least 2 hours.
4. Cut into bars and store in meal prep containers.

16. Mediterranean Chickpea and Quinoa Bowl

Ingredients:

- 1 cup cooked quinoa
- 1 can (15 oz) chickpeas, drained and rinsed
- 1 cup cucumber, diced
- 1 cup cherry tomatoes, halved
- 1/4 cup red onion, finely chopped
- 2 tablespoons fresh basil, chopped
- 2 tablespoons extra virgin olive oil

- Juice of 1 lemon

- Salt and pepper to taste

Method:

1. In a bowl, combine cooked quinoa, chickpeas, cucumber, cherry tomatoes, red onion, and fresh basil.
2. In a separate small bowl, whisk together olive oil, lemon juice, salt, and pepper to create the dressing.
3. Drizzle the dressing over the bowl's contents and toss well.
4. Divide into meal prep containers and refrigerate.

17. Turmeric and Ginger Carrot Soup

Ingredients:

- 2 cups carrots, peeled and chopped

- 1 small onion, chopped

- 2 cloves garlic, minced

- 1 teaspoon ground turmeric

- 1/2 teaspoon ground ginger

- 4 cups vegetable broth

- 1 tablespoon olive oil

- Salt and pepper to taste

- Fresh cilantro for garnish (optional)

Method:

1. Heat olive oil in a large pot over medium heat.

2. Add chopped onion and garlic, sauté until fragrant.

3. Add chopped carrots, ground turmeric, and ground ginger. Sauté for a few more minutes.

4. Pour in vegetable broth, bring to a boil, then reduce heat and simmer until the carrots are tender (about 20 25 minutes).

5. Use an immersion blender to blend the soup until smooth.

6. Season with salt and pepper, garnish with fresh cilantro, and portion into meal prep containers.

18. Mixed Berry Chia Pudding

Ingredients:

- 1/4 cup chia seeds

- 1 cup unsweetened almond milk

- 1/2 cup mixed berries (strawberries, blueberries, raspberries)

- 1 tablespoon honey or maple syrup (optional)

Method:

1. In a jar or container, combine chia seeds and almond milk.

2. Stir well, ensuring the chia seeds are fully submerged.

3. Refrigerate for at least 2 hours or overnight, allowing the chia seeds to absorb the liquid and thicken.

4. Before serving, top with mixed berries and drizzle with honey or maple syrup if desired.

19. Roasted Brussels Sprouts and Butternut Squash

Ingredients:

- 2 cups Brussels sprouts, trimmed and halved
- 2 cups butternut squash, peeled and diced
- 2 tablespoons olive oil
- 1 teaspoon dried thyme
- Salt and pepper to taste
- Balsamic glaze for drizzling (optional)

Method:

1. Preheat your oven to 425°F (220°C).

2. Toss Brussels sprouts and butternut squash with olive oil, dried thyme, salt, and pepper.

3. Spread the mixture on a baking sheet and roast for 20 25 minutes or until the vegetables are tender and slightly caramelized.

4. Drizzle with balsamic glaze if desired and divide into meal prep containers.

20. Green Tea and Ginger Infused Water

Ingredients:

- 4 cups water

- 2 green tea bags

- 1 inch piece of fresh ginger, sliced

- 1 lemon, sliced

- Fresh mint leaves

Method:

1. In a pitcher, steep green tea bags in 4 cups of hot water for
   3 5 minutes.
2. Add sliced ginger, lemon slices, and fresh mint leaves to
   the tea.
3. Allow it to cool and refrigerate.
4. Pour into individual bottles or jars for a refreshing and anti
   inflammatory beverage.

21. Mediterranean Quinoa Salad

Ingredients:

- 1 cup cooked quinoa
- 1/2 cup cucumber, diced
- 1/2 cup cherry tomatoes, halved
- 1/4 cup Kalamata olives, pitted and sliced
- 1/4 cup red onion, finely chopped
- 1/4 cup fresh parsley, chopped
- 2 tablespoons extra virgin olive oil
- Juice of 1 lemon
- 1 teaspoon dried oregano

- Salt and pepper to taste

- Feta cheese crumbles for garnish (optional)

Method:

1. In a bowl, combine cooked quinoa, diced cucumber, cherry tomatoes, Kalamata olives, red onion, and fresh parsley.

2. In a separate small bowl, whisk together olive oil, lemon juice, dried oregano, salt, and pepper to create the dressing.

3. Drizzle the dressing over the salad and toss well.

4. Garnish with feta cheese crumbles before serving.

22. Anti Inflammatory Turmeric Tea

Ingredients:

- 2 cups water

- 1 teaspoon ground turmeric

- 1/2 teaspoon ground ginger

- 1/2 teaspoon ground cinnamon

- 1 teaspoon honey (optional)

- A squeeze of lemon juice (optional)

Method:

1. In a saucepan, bring 2 cups of water to a boil.

2. Stir in ground turmeric, ground ginger, and ground cinnamon.

3. Simmer for 10 minutes, then strain the tea into a cup.

4. Sweeten with honey and add a squeeze of lemon juice if desired.

5. Pour into a thermos or bottle for a soothing and anti inflammatory beverage.

23. Broccoli and Red Lentil Soup

Ingredients:

- 2 cups broccoli florets
- 1 cup red lentils, rinsed and drained
- 1 onion, chopped
- 2 cloves garlic, minced
- 1 teaspoon ground cumin
- 1/2 teaspoon ground coriander
- 6 cups vegetable broth
- 2 tablespoons olive oil

- Salt and pepper to taste

- Fresh cilantro for garnish (optional)

Method:

1. Heat olive oil in a large pot over medium heat.
2. Add chopped onion and garlic, sauté until fragrant.
3. Stir in ground cumin and ground coriander.
4. Add broccoli florets, red lentils, and vegetable broth.
5. Bring to a boil, then reduce heat and simmer for 20 25 minutes until lentils are tender.
6. Use an immersion blender to blend the soup until smooth.
7. Season with salt and pepper, garnish with fresh cilantro, and portion into meal prep containers.

24. Spiced Chickpea and Vegetable Curry

Ingredients:

- 1 can (15 oz) chickpeas, drained and rinsed

- 1 cup cauliflower florets

- 1 cup sweet potato cubes

- 1 cup bell pepper, diced

- 1 onion, chopped

- 2 cloves garlic, minced

- 1 can (15 oz) diced tomatoes

- 2 tablespoons olive oil

- 1 tablespoon curry powder

- 1/2 teaspoon ground turmeric

- Salt and pepper to taste

Method:

1. In a large skillet, heat olive oil over medium heat.

2. Add chopped onion and garlic, sauté until translucent.

3. Stir in curry powder and ground turmeric.

4. Add chickpeas, cauliflower, sweet potato, bell pepper, and diced tomatoes (with their juices).

5. Simmer for 15 20 minutes until the vegetables are tender.

6. Season with salt and pepper.

7. Divide into meal prep containers and refrigerate.

25. Anti Inflammatory Berry Smoothie

Ingredients:

- 1 cup mixed berries (strawberries, blueberries, raspberries)

- 1/2 cup spinach leaves

- 1/2 cup unsweetened almond milk

- 1/2 teaspoon ground turmeric
- 1 tablespoon chia seeds
- 1/2 teaspoon honey (optional)

Method:

1. Blend mixed berries, spinach, almond milk, ground turmeric, chia seeds, and honey (if desired) until smooth.
2. Pour into individual bottles or jars for a nutrient packed and anti inflammatory breakfast or snack.

26. Lemon Garlic Shrimp and Asparagus

Ingredients:

- 8 oz shrimp, peeled and deveined
- 1 bunch asparagus, trimmed
- 2 tablespoons olive oil
- 2 cloves garlic, minced
- Zest and juice of 1 lemon
- Salt and pepper to taste
- Fresh parsley for garnish (optional)

Method:

1. Preheat your oven to 425°F (220°C).

2. In a bowl, combine shrimp, trimmed asparagus, olive oil, minced garlic, lemon zest, lemon juice, salt, and pepper.

3. Spread the mixture on a baking sheet and roast for 10 12 minutes until shrimp are pink and cooked through.

4. Garnish with fresh parsley and divide into meal prep containers.

27. Cabbage and Kale Slaw

Ingredients:

- 2 cups shredded green cabbage
- 2 cups chopped kale
- 1/4 cup grated carrot
- 1/4 cup sliced red onion
- 1/4 cup sliced almonds
- 2 tablespoons extra virgin olive oil
- Juice of 1 lime
- 1 teaspoon honey or maple syrup (optional)
- Salt and pepper to taste

Method:

1. In a large bowl, combine shredded green cabbage, chopped kale, grated carrot, sliced red onion, and sliced almonds.
2. In a separate small bowl, whisk together olive oil, lime juice, honey or maple syrup (if desired), salt, and pepper to create the dressing.
3. Drizzle the dressing over the slaw and toss well.
4. Portion into meal prep containers and refrigerate.

28. Turmeric and Ginger Baked Chicken

Ingredients:

- 4 boneless, skinless chicken breasts
- 1 tablespoon olive oil
- 1 teaspoon ground turmeric
- 1/2 teaspoon ground ginger
- 2 cloves garlic, minced
- Salt and pepper to taste
- Lemon wedges for garnish

Method:

1. Preheat your oven to 375°F (190°C).
2. In a bowl, combine olive oil, ground turmeric, ground ginger, minced garlic, salt, and pepper.
3. Rub the mixture over chicken breasts.
4. Place the chicken in a baking dish and bake for 25 30 minutes or until the chicken reaches an internal temperature of 165°F (74°C).
5. Garnish with lemon wedges and divide into meal prep containers.

29. Anti Inflammatory Berry Chia Jam

Ingredients:

- 2 cups mixed berries (strawberries, blueberries, raspberries)
- 2 tablespoons chia seeds
- 1 tablespoon honey or maple syrup (optional)

Method:

1. In a saucepan, heat mixed berries over low heat, mashing them with a fork or potato masher.
2. Stir in chia seeds and honey or maple syrup (if desired).
3. Continue cooking for 10 15 minutes until the mixture thickens.
4. Let it cool and divide into small jars for a healthy and homemade berry jam.

30. Spinach and Feta Stuffed Chicken Breast

Ingredients:

- 4 boneless, skinless chicken breasts
- 2 cups fresh spinach leaves
- 1/2 cup crumbled feta cheese
- 2 cloves garlic, minced
- 1 tablespoon olive oil
- Salt and pepper to taste
- Toothpicks

Method:

1. Preheat your oven to 375°F (190°C).

2. In a skillet, heat olive oil over medium heat.

3. Add minced garlic and sauté for 30 seconds.

4. Add fresh spinach and cook until wilted.

5. Butterfly each chicken breast and stuff with wilted spinach and crumbled feta cheese.

6. Secure with toothpicks and place in a baking dish.

7. Season with salt and pepper, then bake for 25 30 minutes or until the chicken is cooked through.

8. Remove toothpicks before dividing into meal prep containers.

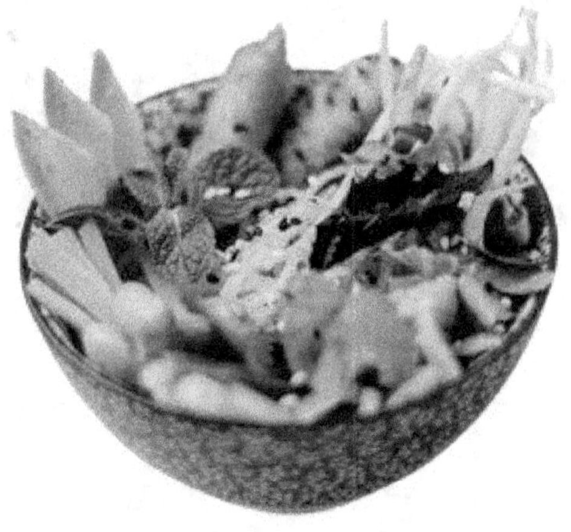

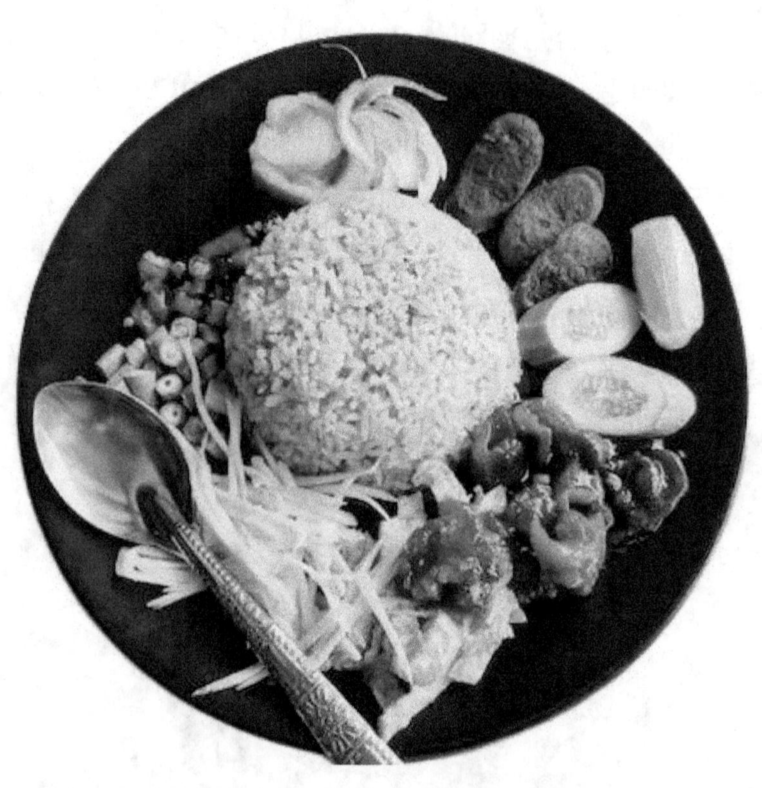

CONCLUSION

In our journey through this Anti Inflammatory Diet Meal Prep Cookbook, we've embarked on a path to transform our lives through the power of food.

We've learned that the journey to optimal health is not just about what we eat; it's about how we eat and how we take charge of our well being.

Within these pages, we've explored a myriad of recipes that tantalize the taste buds while promoting inflammation fighting nutrients.

We've discovered that anti inflammatory eating isn't merely a diet but a lifestyle, a commitment to nourishing our bodies with the best nature has to offer.

Yet, it's not just about the recipes; it's about the profound impact they can have on our health. We've witnessed how thoughtful meal preparation can lead to increased energy, reduced pain, enhanced mental clarity, and a strengthened immune system.

But this journey doesn't end with the last page. It's a lifelong commitment to wellness, a promise to ourselves to choose health and vitality every day.

It's about recognizing that our bodies are remarkable, and they respond positively when we treat them with kindness and respect.

As you take the knowledge and recipes from this cookbook into your daily life, remember that you have the power to shape your health destiny.

Cherish your body, savor your meals, and relish the journey towards a vibrant, inflammation free life.

May these recipes and insights continue to inspire you on your path to better health, proving that delicious, healing, and nourishing meals are within reach, one mindful bite at a time.

Your health is your greatest wealth, and you now hold the keys to unlock its full potential.

Embrace it, celebrate it, and thrive in it.